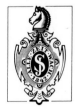

Klaus Johansen   Sam Dagogo-Jack

Diabetes
Guide

With 12 Figures and 47 Tables

Springer-Verlag
Berlin Heidelberg New York
London Paris Tokyo
Hong Kong Barcelona
Budapest

Klaus Johansen, M.D.
Department of Medicine
Sct. Hans Hospital
4000 Roskilde, Denmark

Sam Dagogo-Jack, M.D.
Metabolism Division
Washington University
School of Medicine
660 South Euclid Avenue
St. Louis, Missouri 63110
U.S.A.

ISBN 3-540-54429-1 Springer-Verlag Berlin Heidelberg New York
ISBN 0-387-54429-1 Springer-Verlag New York Berlin Heidelberg

Library of Congress Cataloging-in-Publication Data
Johansen, Klaus. Diabetes guide / Klaus Johansen, Sam Dagogo-Jack.   p.   cm.
Includes bibliographical references and indexes.
ISBN 3-540-54429-1 (Springer-Verlag Berlin Heidelberg New York). –
ISBN 0-387-54429-1 (Springer-Verlag New York Berlin Heidelberg)
1. Diabetes––Handbooks, manuals, etc.   I. Dagogo-Jack, Sam, 1954–   II. Title.
RC660.J52   1992   616.4'62––dc20   91-37275

Typesetting: Elsner & Behrens GmbH, Oftersheim
Printing and binding: Druckhaus Beltz, Hemsbach/Bergstr.
27/3145 - 5 4 3 2 1 0 – Printed on acid-free paper

Our main business in life is not to see what lies dimly at a distance, but to do what lies clearly at hand.

Thomas Carlyle

Preface

There is already abundant information on the theoretical and practical aspects of diabetes in various standard textbooks and monographs. However, new information is also continually being added to our knowledge of diabetes by the proliferation of articles in specialized journals.

The aim of DIABETES GUIDE is to epitomize the current knowledge on diabetes and present it in an easily digestible format.

By using tables, diagrams, curves, and flow charts to present practical state-of-the-art recommendations, we have reduced verbiage to a minimum in this ready-reference guide for physicians, nurses, dietitians and all others who are involved in the care of diabetic patients. Practising physicians and those training for higher diplomas and fellowships in diabetes and endocrinology should find the tabulated, rather than textual, approach particularly useful. The treatment recommendations in some instances represent, in the authors' opinion, the best of several options. Treatment of the individual patient is, of course, best individualized but we believe that the information presented here will provide the reader with a suitable basis for tailoring care of each diabetic patient.

KLAUS JOHANSEN
SAM DAGOGO-JACK

Contents

General Information

Definition of Diabetes Mellitus

Untreated diabetes mellitus (DM) is characterized by hyperglycaemia and other biochemical abnormalities resulting from absolute or relative insulin deficiency.

The diabetic has a long-term risk of developing progressive microangiopathy of the retina, kidney and nerves and aggravated atherosclerosis (macroangiopathy).

Classification of Diabetes Mellitus and Allied Categories of Glucose Intolerance[1]

Clinical Classes

Diabetes mellitus

    Insulin-dependent diabetes mellitus (IDDM)
    Non-insulin-dependent diabetes mellitus (NIDDM)
        Non-obese
        Obese

---

[1] WHO (1985) Diabetes mellitus: report of a WHO study group. WHO, Geneva, (Technical report series 727).

Malnutrition-related diabetes mellitus (MRDM)
Other types of diabetes associated with certain conditions and syndromes, including: pancreatic disease, disease of hormonal aetiology, drug- or chemical-induced conditions, abnormalities of insulin or its receptors, certain genetic syndromes
Impaired glucose tolerance (IGT)

> Non-obese
> Obese
> Associated with certain conditions and syndromes

Gestational diabetes

Statistical Risk Classes
(Subjects with Normal Glucose Tolerance but Substantially Increased Risk of Developing Diabetes)

Previous abnormality of glucose tolerance
Potential abnormality of glucose tolerance

Malnutrition-Related Diabetes Mellitus (Tropical Diabetes)[2]

Protein-Deficient Pancreatic Diabetes (PDPD)

Diagnostic Criteria
Blood glucose >11.1 mmol/l
Onset <30 years of age
Body mass index [weight (kg)/height^2 (m)] <19
Non-ketosis prone
Undernutrition
Insulin requirement >60 units/day or >1.5 units/kg

---

[2] Ahuja MM (1980) Diabetes-Special Problems in Developing Countries Bull Deliv Health Care Dev Countries 1:5–6.

Fibrocalculous Pancreatic Diabetes (FCPD)

Diagnostic Criteria
As for PDPD plus:
Recurrent abdominal pain
Pancreatic calcification
Abscence of alcoholism, gall stones or hyperparathyroidism

Countries Affected[3]

PDPD and FCPD	FCPD only	PDPD only
India	Brazil	Tanzania
Thailand	Madagascar	Kenya
Jamaica	Zimbabwe	Papua New Guinea
Indonesia		Malaysia
Borneo		Brunei
New Guinea		Nauru
Zaire		Fiji
Ivory Coast		
Ghana		
Benin		
Togo		
Nigeria		
Cameroon		
South Africa		

[3] WHO (1985) Diabetes mellitus: report of a WHO study group. WHO, Geneva, (Technical report series 727).

Clinical and Biochemical Characteristics of Malnutrition-Related Diabetes Mellitus

	PDPD	FCPD
History of malnutrition	Invariable	Common
Malnutrition on presentation	Common	Common
Poor socio-economic status	Common	Common
Cassava consumption	$\pm$	Common
Age at onset (years)	10–40	15–35
Sex	M>F	M>F
Ketosis	None?	Uncommon
Insulin requirements	<1.3–2 units/kg	Moderate to high
Exocrine pancreatic malfunction	Rare	Common
Abdominal pain	Rare	Common
Pancreatic calcification	Absent	Common
Pancreatic fibrosis	Occurs	Invariably
C-peptide secretion	Present	Generally present
Islet cell antibodies	Absent	Absent
HLA association	None	None
Microangiopathy	Common	Common
Neuropathy	Very common	Very common
Macroangiopathy	Rare	Rare

Prevalence of Insulin-Dependent Diabetes Mellitus in Certain Populations, 1970–1980

Location	Age group (years)	Methods	Prevalence
UK	0–26	National survey of health and development	3.40
Scandinavia	0–14	National registry and hospital records	0.83–2.23
USA	5–17	School records	1.93
France	0–19	Central registry	0.32
Cuba	0–15	National registry	0.14
China	10–19	Survey	0.09
Japan	7–15	School records	0.07

Incidence of Insulin-Dependent Diabetes Mellitus[4]

Location	Period	Age group (years)	Incidence per 100000 person · years at risk
Sweden (North)	1973–77	0–14	38
Finland	1970–79	0–19	27
Pittsburg, USA	1965–76	0–19	10–16
Rhode Island, USA	1979–80	0–29	14
Scotland	1968–76	0–18	14
Netherlands	1978–80	0–19	11
Toronto, Canada	1976–80	0–18	9
Israel			
Ashkenazim	1975–80	0–20	6.3
Non-Ashkenazim	1975–80	0–20	2.6

[4] WHO (1985) Diabetes mellitus: report of a WHO study group. WHO, Geneva, (Technical report series 727).

Characteristic Differences Between Insulin-Dependent and Non-Insulin-Dependent Diabetes Mellitus

Thin, ketosis-prone	Obese, ketosis-resistant
Insulin required for survival	Often treatable by diet or drugs
Onset predomiantly in childhood and early adulthood	Onset predominantly after age 40
Less than 50% concordance in monozygotic twins	Close to 100% concordance in monozygotic twins
Flat insulin response to a glucose load	Variable insulin response
Associated with other autoimmune endocrinopathies	Not associated with other autoimmune endocrinopathies
HLA association	No HLA association
Seasonal variation in incidence	No seasonal variation in incidence

Diagnosis of Diabetes Based on Nonstandardized Blood Glucose Values[5]

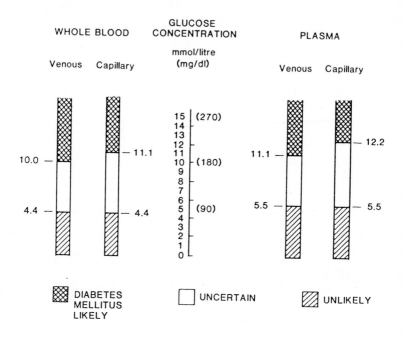

Procedure for Oral Glucose Tolerance Test

Should be performed in the morning

At least 3 days of unrestricted diet (>150 g carbohydrate daily) and usual physical activity

Preceded by an overnight fast of 10–16 h (water allowed)

---

[5] WHO (1985) Diabetes mellitus: report of a WHO study group. WHO, Geneva, (Technical report series 727).

Smoking is not permitted during the test

Exclude medications, inactivity, infection

Give 75 g glucose in 250–300 ml water over the course of 5 min; children 1.75 g/kg body weight

Draw blood samples fasting and 2 h after the test load

Use specific enzymatic glucose method

Diagnostic Values for Oral Glucose Tolerance Test[6]

	Glucose concentration (mmol/l)			
	Whole blood		Plasma	
	Venous	Capillary	Venous	Capillary
Diabetes mellitus				
Fasting	≥ 6.7	≥ 6.7	≥ 7.8	≥ 7.8
2 h after glucose load	≥10.0	≥11.1	≥11.1	≥12.2
Impaired glucose tolerance				
Fasting	< 6.7	< 6.7	< 7.8	> 7.8
2 h after glucose load	6.7–10.0	7.8–11.1	7.8–11.1	8.9–12.2

[6] WHO (1985) Diabetes mellitus: report of a WHO Study Group. WHO, Geneva, (Technical report series 727).

Conditions and Syndromes Associated with Glucose Intolerance

Fever
Physical inactivity
Prolonged fast
Low carbohydrate intake
Pregnancy
Obesity
Malnutrition
Acute and chronic disease
Endocrinopathies (see below)
Diffuse pancreatic disorders
Insulin receptor abnormalities
Genetic and chromosomal syndromes
Drugs: Thiazides, glucocorticoids, oestrogens, benzodiazepines, morphine, alcohol, clonidine, indomethacin

Endocrinopathies Associated with Glucose Intolerance

Acromegaly
Sexual ateliotic dwarfism
Hyperprolactinaemia
Cushing's syndrome
Pheochromocytoma
Primary hyperaldosteronism
Hyperthyroidism
Hypothyroidism
Disorders of calcium and phosporous metabolism
Glucagonoma
Somatostatinoma
Gastrinoma

Vipoma
Carcinoid syndrome
Multiple endocrine neoplasia

Symptoms and Disorders Indicating Examination for Diabetes Mellitus

Polyuria, polydipsia, weight loss
Genital pruritus, balanitis, furunculosis
Blurred vision, paraesthesias, paresis
Glycosuria
Obesity
Pregnancy
Previous high-birth-weight infants
Previous reduced glucose tolerance
Atherosclerosis
Hyperlipoproteinaemia

History and Physical Examination of Diabetic Patients

The medical record is a normal medical record with special emphasis on the following:

History

Family history: Diabetes and other endocrine diseases, especially thyroid and adrenal
Start of diabetes: Age, symptoms, treatment, admissions
Past history: Hyper- and hypoglycaemic symptoms, treatment

11

Symptoms of long-term diabetic complications: visual disturbances, impotence, gastrointestinal symptoms, bladder dysfunction, decreased sensation, numbness, angina pectoris, intermittent claudication, foot ulcers
Medication: Insulin dose, dose of oral antidiabetic drugs, interactions
Tobacco, alcohol: Amount
Diet: History
Self-care: Methods, frequency, record kept?
Physical exercise: Degree, frequency
Social conditions: Who prepares the diet? Who injects the insulin? Does the patient live alone?

Physical Examination

Look especially for: Rubeosis faciei, cataract, skin carbuncles, granuloma annulare, necrobiosis, shin spots, injection pads, acetone foetor, Kussmaul respiration, dehydration, raised blood pressure, decreased or absent peripheral pulses, deep tendon reflexes, and vibratory perception, retinopathy, stiff-hand syndrome, Dupuytren's contracture

Self-Care

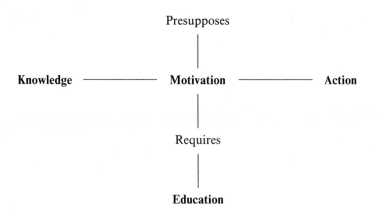

Self-Monitoring

NIDDM Patients, Uncontrolled

Daily measurement of urine glucose in first morning urine, plus 2 h after a meal until glycosuria $< 1/2\%$. If glycosuria is $> 3\%$ (167 mmol/l), blood glucose should be measured daily in the fasting state and $1\frac{1}{2}$ h after a meal.

NIDDM Patients, Well-Controlled

Urine glucose twice weekly 2 h after a meal.

NIDDM Patients, Insulin-Treated

As for IDDM patients.

IDDM Patients, Uncontrolled

Measure blood glucose (fingerstick) in the fasting state, about $1\frac{1}{2}$ h after breakfast, lunch, and dinner, and at 23.00 hours. Do 2–3 times weekly until "good control" has been achieved. Check urine for ketone bodies morning and evening.

IDDM Patients, Well-Controlled

Blood glucose in the fasting state, $1\frac{1}{2}$ h after breakfast, lunch and dinner, and at 23.00 hours once weekly.

Indications

Intensive insulin therapy with insulin pump or pen
Pregnancy
Hypoglycaemia-prone patients
Illnesses
Unreliable urine glucose monitoring
Special circumstances: renal dialysis, nocturnal hypoglycaemia, physical training/competition

Renal Threshold for Glucose

Definition: The lowest blood glucose concentration at which glucose occurs in urine.

The renal threshold for glucose varies individually from approximately 5 to 15 mmol/l with a mean around 10 mmol/l.

Measurement of urine glucose is easy, cheap and non invasive.

Urine glucose does not reflect the ambient blood glucose concentration but gives a retrospective index of the blood glucose concentration in the period the urine is produced and stored in the bladder.

Measurement of glycosuria obviously does not give information about blood glucose levels below the renal threshold and can therefore not be used in hypoglycaemic and normoglycaemic patients.

The renal threshold for glucose increases with age and decreases during pregnancy.

Glycated Haemoglobin

Glycated haemoglobin (Hba_{1c}) expressed as a percentage of the total haemoglobin gives a cumulative index of the mean blood glucose level over the preceding 6–8 weeks.

The rate of glycation is related to blood glucose concentration by irreversible non-enzymatic process.

Severe anaemia, pregnancy, renal failure, and haemoglobinopathies influence the estimate.

Reference ranges should be established and calibration of raised HbA_{1c} values against the corresponding degrees of hyperglycaemia should be established.

With most methods, proportions of HbA_{1c} exceeding 8%–9% of the total haemoglobin are abnormal. An excess of 12% or more indicates severe and sustained hyperglycaemia.

HbA_{1c} is an objective measure which does not require the patient to be cooperative. It is unaffected by meals, exercise or time of drawing. It gives the degree of regulation in a single figure.

It is a retrospective measure and it does not signify therapeutic changes. HbA_{1c} does not reflect hypoglycaemic episodes.

Measurement of HbA_{1c} three to four times yearly gives a valuable integrated picture of the degree of diabetes control.

References ranges differ between laboratories.

Mean blood glucose from the last 6–8 weeks can be estimated roughly from HbA_{1c} by the equation:[7]

$$\text{Mean blood glucose} = (HbA_{1c} \times 33.3) - 86$$

---

[7] Nathan DM (1984) "Glycosylated hemoglobin; what it is and how to use it" New Engl J Med 310:341–46.

Non-enzymatic Glycation of Haemoglobin

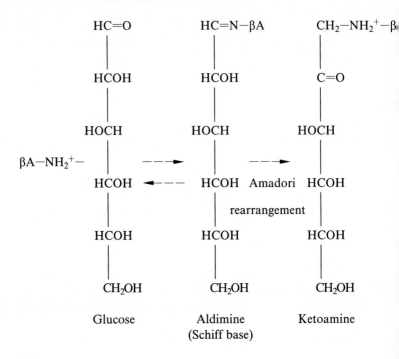

βA−NH₂ = Haemoglobin molecule (β chain)

Fructosamine

Like haemoglobin, serum proteins can be glycated by non-enzymatic reactions. "Fructosamine" is a generally accepted term for the ketoamines formed by this reaction.

Estimation of fructosamine gives an integrated expression of the blood glucose level during the last 2–3 weeks.

Estimation of the Endogenous Insulin Secretion Using the C-Peptide Concentration

Type of patient State	C-peptide concentration (approx.) (nmol/l)
Non-diabetic, NIDDM	
Fasting	>0.3
After glucagon 1 mg IV	>0.6
IDDM	
Fasting	<0.3
After glucagon 1 mg IV	<0.6

Clinical Application of the C-Peptide Assay

Condition	C-peptide
Acute diabetes	Decreased to absent
Chronic insulin-deficient diabetes	Absent
Diabetes in remission	Increases in response to glucagon and glucose
Endogenous hyperinsulinaemia in diabetic patients	No suppression during hypoglycaemia
Insulinoma	No suppression during hypoglycaemia
Factitious hypoglycaemia	Suppressed
Hypoglycaemia due to spontaneous insulin antibodies	Suppressed

Investigation of Long-Term Diabetic Patients

Examinations are performed at diagnosis, p.r.n. and:

Ophthalmoscopy, vision	In IDDM, once a year after the first 5 years. In NIDDM, once a year after the first 2 years
Blood pressure	Every 3 months
Serum creatinine	In case of intermittent or persistent macroalbuminuria every 3 months
Urine microscopy, culture	Once a year in case of intermittent or constant macroalbuminuria or cystopathy
Proteinuria	See diabetic nephropathy (p. 91)
Foot pulses, reflexes, vibratory perception, sensitivity	Once a year and in case of previous foot ulcers at every examination
Lipid profile	Once a year but more frequently during treatment of hyperlipidaemia
ECG	When cardiopulmonary symptoms are present
Height in children	Once a year until growth has stopped
Chest X-ray	At diagnosis and in event of cardiorespiratory illness

Pancreatic Transplantation –
Patient and Graft Functional Survival Rates at 1 Year,
University of Minnesota (1984–1988)[8]

Category	Patient survival (%)	Graft survival (%)
Pancreas plus kidney	91	71
Pancreas after kidney	87	47
Pancreas alone	96	48

Therapeutic Goals

Fasting blood glucose <7 mmol/l
Postprandial blood glucose <11 mmol/l
No blood glucose values <3 mmol/l
Glycated haemoglobin (HbA$_{1c}$) $<8\%$
No ketonuria
Albuminuria <30 mg/24 h
Serum total cholesterol <6.5 mmol/l
Serum high-density lipoprotein (HDL) cholesterol >0.9 mmol/l
Fasting triglyceride <2.2 mmol/l
Physical and psychosocial well-being
Normal body weight and normal growth of children
Blood pressure $<140/90$ mmHg (young) and $<160/95$ mmHg (old)

---

[8] For details of protocols see: Sutherland DER, Goetz FC, Moudry KC et al. (1988) Pancreatic transplantation – a single institutions experience. Diab Nutr Metab 1:57–66.

19

Diet

Energy Requirements

Factors for calculation of 24-h energy requirement for children and adults with various levels of physical activity

	Age (years)	Activity		
		Low	Mean	High
Children	1– 3	350	400	450
	4– 6	300	350	400
	7–10	275	350	400
Males	11–14	225	250	275
	15–18	175	200	225
	19–22	150	175	200
	23–50	125	150	175
	51–70	110	125	150
	71	100	110	125
Females	11–14	150	175	200
	15–18	135	150	175
	19–22	120	135	150
	23–50	110	120	135
	51–70	100	110	120
	71	95	100	110

Energy requirement = Ideal body weight $\times$ factor
Ideal body weight = Males: [[Height (cm)] $-$ 100] $-$ 10% = kg
Females: [[[Height (cm)] $-$ 100] $-$ 10%] $-$ 3 = kg
kcal = kJ/4.2.

Protein, Fat, Carbohydrate and Energy Content of Some Common Food Items

Food item (100 g)	Protein (g)	Fat (g)	Carbo-hydrate (g)	Energy (kJ)
Chicken, roasted with skin, light meat	29	11	0	932
Pork, lean	29	9	0	840
Veal, rump, lean	32	2	0	655
Beef, lean	34	7	0	924
Lamb, leg, lean	29	6	0	735
Herring, fresh, broiled	24	16	0	650
Cod, broiled	27	5	0	714
Plaice	17	2	0	375
Vegetables, mean	2	0	5	105
Carrots, raw	1	0	10	176
Potatoes, no skin, boiled	2	0	15	273
Fruit, mean	1	0	15	252
Bread, white	9	4	49	1110
Egg, 50 g	6	6	0	325
Milk, whole (3.7%)	3	4	5	270
Milk, low fat (1%)	3	1	5	179
Milk, skimmed	4	5	0	151
Yoghurt, whole	3	3	4	256
Butter	0	81	0	3024
Margarine	0	76	0	2856
Cream, medium (25%)	3	25	3	1037
Cream, light	3	19	4	811
Cream, whipping, heavy	2	37	3	1457
Cheese (45%)	25	28	1	1499
Cheese (20%)	11	8	5	580

Recommended Carbohydrate, Protein and Fat Contents of a Diabetic Diet

	% of energy content
Carbohydrate	55–65
Protein	10–15
Fat	30

The ratio saturated, monounsaturated and polyunsaturated fatty acids should be 1:1 $^2/_3$ and the cholesterol intake <300 mg/day.

Recommended Amounts of Absorbable and Non-absorbable Carbohydrates in the Diabetic Diet

Type of carbohydrate	Amount (weight %)
Absorbable	
Monosaccharides: glucose, fructose, galactose	⎫
Disaccharides: maltose, lactose, saccharose	⎬ 20
Oligosaccharides: syrups	⎭
Polysaccharides: starch, glycogen	65
Non-absorbable	
Oligosaccharides: hexose, e.g. stachyose in soyabeans	⎫
Polysaccharides	⎬
Water-soluble: e.g. pectin in apples and galacto-mannans in leguminous fruits and vegetables	⎬ 5
Water-insoluble: e.g. hemicellulose and cellulose	10

Characteristics of a High-Fibre Diet

Beneficial Effects

Delayed gastric emptying
Prolonged intestinal transit (depends on fibre constituents)
Decreased glucose, cholesterol and triglyceride absorption
Reduced insulin and sulphonylurea requirements

Adverse Effects

Flatulence, abdominal discomfort
Increased defaecation, diarrhoea
Phytobezoar formation with gastric hypotony
Potential for loss of vitamins or minerals

Alcoholic Beverages

Beverage	Serv-ving (ml)	Alcohol (g)	Carbo-hydrate (g)	Energy (kJ)
Beer				
Regular	360	13.0	13.7	634
Light	360	10.1	6.0	378
Distilled				
Gin, Rum, Vodka, Whisky	45	15.3	trace	449
Cognac	30	10.7	trace	315
Wines				
Red/rose	120	11.6	1.0	357
Dry white	120	11.3	0.4	336
Sweet white	120	11.8	4.9	428
Sparkling	120	11.9	3.6	412

Beverage	Serving (ml)	Alcohol (g)	Carbohydrate (g)	Energy (kJ)
Appetizers/desert wines				
Dry sherry	60	9.4	1.5	307
Sweet sherry, port	60	9.4	7.0	395
Vermouth, dry	90	12.6	4.2	441
Vermouth, sweet	90	12.2	13.9	592

Artificial Sweeteners

	Relative-sweetness in comparison with sugar	Contains calories	Tolerates boiling	Disadvantages	Usability for diabetics
Cyclamate	Somewhat more	No	Yes	None	Unlimited
Saccharin	300×	No	Yes	Bitter aftertaste	Unlimited
Aspartame	200×	No	No	None	Unlimited
Acesulfame-K	200×	No	Yes	None	Unlimited
Sorbitol	½×	Yes	Yes	Laxative	Small amounts
Fructose	1½×	Yes	Yes	None	Small amounts
Xylitol	½×	Yes	Yes	Laxative	Small amounts

Energy Requirements During Various Activities

Low (420–840 kJ/h)	Moderate (840–1470 kJ/h)	High (1680–3780 kJ/h)
Driving a car	Moderate housework	Manual labour
Fishing	Bicycling	Wood chopping
Laboratory work	Bowling	Aerobic exercise
Light housework	Brisk walking	Dancing (fast)
Secretarial work	Dancing (slow)	Ice skating
Teaching	Factory work	Running
Walking casually	Gardening	Soccer
	Golf	Climbing
	Roller skating	Other outdoor sports
	Truck driving	Tennis (singles)

Slimming Advice

Eat less
Eat three main meals and three snacks every day
Keep fixed meal times
Eat fibre-containing bread
Eat vegetables at all meals
Eat slowly and chew thoroughly
Avoid alcohol
Do more exercise
Check your weight once a week

Body Mass Index

Body mass index (BMI) = Weight (kg)/Height^2 (m)

>30 = obese
$25-30$ = overweight
<25 = acceptable

Glycaemic Index

Definition: The blood glucose rise after the food item under investigation, expressed as a percentage of the blood glucose rise after a standard meal with the same amount of digestible carbohydrate.

Calculation: Blood glucose rise (area under the curve) after the meal under investigation, divided by the blood glucose rise (area under the curve) after the standard meal.

The glycaemic index gives an indication of the blood glucose level after intake of different food items.

Insulin-Dependent Diabetes Mellitus

Biochemistry of Insulin Deficiency

(Figure see p. 30/31)

1, glucokinase
2, glucose-6-phosphatase
3, phosphoglucoisomerase
4, fructose-1,6-diphosphatase
5, 6-phosphofructokinase
6, fructoaldolase
7, trioseisomerase
8, phosphoenolpyruvate carboxykinase
9, pyruvate kinase
10, pyruvate carboxylase
11, lactate dehydrogenase
12, pyruvate dehydrogenase
13, pyruvate carboxylase
14, isocitrate dehydrogenase
15, α-ketoglutarate dehydrogenase
16, citrate cleavage enzyme
17, acetyl-CoA carboxylase
18, fatty acid synthase
19, glycerol phosphate acyltransferase
20, hormone-sensitive lipase
21, hydroxymethylglutaryl-CoA reductase
22, glycogen synthase
23, glycogen phosphorylase

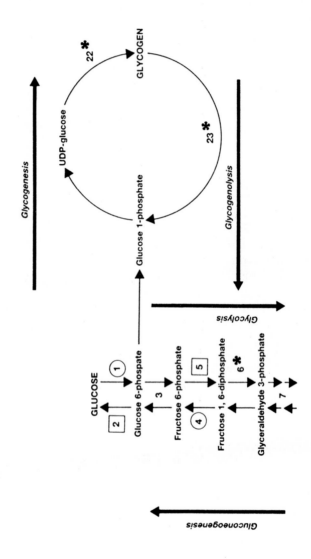

30

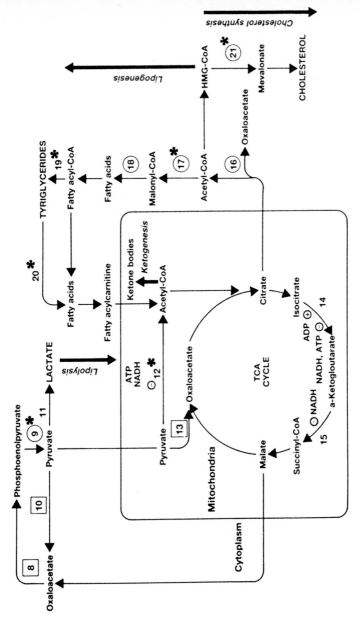

31

Asterisk indicate interconvertible enzymes that are phosphorylated or dephosphorylated depending on the ratio of insulin to glucagon. *UDP,* uridine diphosphate; *HMG-Coa,* hydroxymethylglutaryl-CoAM; *ATP,* adenosine triphosphate; *NADH,* nicotinamide adenine dinucleotide (reduced form); *TCA,* tricarboxyclic acid; *ADP,* adenosine diphosphate

Physiology of Insulin Deficiency

Physiology	Blood and urine chemistry	Symptoms and signs
Glucose uptake (muscle, fat, liver) Gluconeogenesis (liver)	Hyperglycaemia Glycated Hb Glycosuria Osmotic diuresis	Thirst Polydipsia Polyuria Weight loss Polyphagia Tiredness Dehydration
Lipolysis (fat)	Plasma and urine FFA, Acetoacetate, β-Hydroxybutyrate, and Acetone Metabolic acidosis	Kussmaul respiration Acetone foetor Coma

Hb, haemoglobin; FFA, free fatty acids.

Structure of Human Insulin

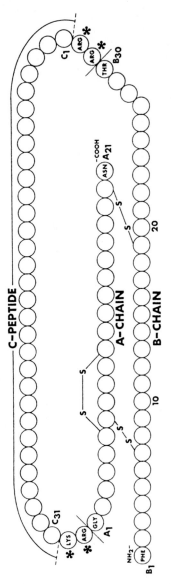

The insulin gene is located on the short arm of chromosome 11. The insulin gene is shown with each of three classes of alleles at the flanking polymorphic region. Also shown are relevant restriction enzyme sites and their coordinates (the 5′-nucleotide of the recognition sequence) relative to the 5′-end of the structural portion of the insulin gene – the start of the insulin messenger RNA (mRNA) transcription. The 1430-base pair *(bp)* insulin gene contains two intervening sequences (introns) of 179 and 786 bp.

Structure of the Insulin Gene

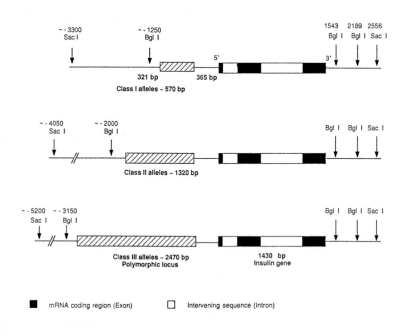

Risk Factors

Genetic (including HLA) (see p. 113)
Islet cell antibodies (islet cell cytoplasmic antibodies, ICA; and islet cell surface antibodies, ICSA)
Viruses
Chemicals

Main Types of Insulin

	Start of effect after (h)	Maximum effect after (h)	Duration of effects (h)

Rapid action
    Regular, soluble,
    crystalline, neutral
	½	2–3	7

Intermediate action Isophane, NPH	1½–2	4–8	12–24

Slow action
    Insulin-zink
    suspension,
    crystalline
	4	10–30	36–72

Intermediate + rapid action	½	4–8	12–24

NPH, neutral protamine Hagedorn.

Insulin Treatment Regimens (One or Two Doses)

1. Single pre-breakfast injection of intermediate-acting insulin. Start with 20 units and increase dose every 3 days depending on blood glucose response to maximally 40 units.
2. High late morning blood glucose: Single pre-breakfast injection of intermediate- and short-acting insulin; two-thirds of morning dose as intermediate-acting, one-third as short-acting. Increase dose depending on blood glucose response to maximally 40 units.
3. High early morning blood glucose: Pre-breakfast and pre-dinner injection of intermediate-acting insulin; two-thirds of total insulin dose given pre-breakfast.
4. High early morning, high late morning and high evening blood glucose: Two doses of intermediate- and short-acting insulin; pre-breakfast injection of two-thirds of total daily dose, one-third daily dose pre-dinner.
5. High afternoon blood glucose: One pre-breakfast dose of inter-mediate- (two-thirds) and short-acting insulin (one-third), one pre-dinner dose of short-acting insulin and bedtime dose of intermediate-acting insulin; two-thirds of total daily dose is given pre-breakfast.
6. High afternoon and evening blood glucose: One pre-breakfast dose of intermediate- or long-acting and short-acting insulin, plus short-acting insulin $\frac{1}{2}$h before lunch and dinner.
7. High early and late morning blood glucose, high afternoon blood glucose, high evening blood glucose: Short-acting insulin $\frac{1}{2}$h before each meal and a dose of intermediate- or long-acting insulin at bedtime.

As a rule of thumb, 25% of the total daily dose is given before breakfast, 15% before lunch, and 20% before dinner as fast-acting insulin. 40% of the total dose is given as intermediate-acting insulin before bedtime. The amount of insulin in each injection will, however, depend on the calorie and carbohydrate content of the meal.

Treatment with multiple insulin injections has become easier with the introduction of insulin injectors (insulin pens).

Insulin effect

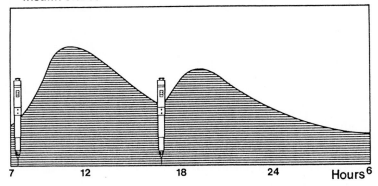

⊟ fast-acting insulin

Insulin effect

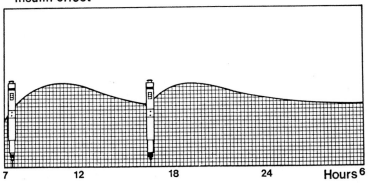

▨ intermediate-acting insulin

Insulin effect

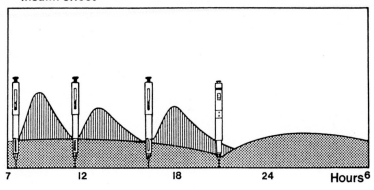

▥ fast-acting insulin, ▨ intermediate-acting insulin

Sliding Scale of Insulin Required to Correct Severe Malregulation

Blood glucose concentration (mmol/l)	Insulin dose required IV (guideline) (units/h)
> 28	6
17–28	4
11–17	3
9–11	2
7–9	1$\frac{1}{2}$
4–7	1
< 4	$\frac{1}{2}$

Measure blood glucose STATIM every hour

Insulin Treatment at Home During Fever Periods

Increase insulin dose by approximately 25% per 1°C over 37.5°C
Measure blood glucose and ketones in urine every 3–4 h
In case of ketonuria and hyperglycaemia inject fast-acting insulin SC
8–12 units STATIM
If no effect, call your doctor
Repeat insulin injections until there is not ketonuria
Continue to monitor blood glucose and urine ketones during the fever
period

Factors Influencing Insulin Absorption and Bioavailability

Injection site and depth
Absorption rate
Insulin concentration and dose
Species source
Insulin antibodies
Ambient blood glucose concentration
Mixtures with modified insulins
Physiological degradation of insulin at injection site
Intrapatient variation in insulin pharmacokinetics

Conversion from Picomoles to Nanograms to Units of Human Insulin, C-Peptide and Proinsulin

Insulin: 5807 dalton

1 pmol	=	5.807 ng
1 ng	=	0.1722 pmol
1 µU	=	0.00615 pmol
28 µU	=	1 ng

C peptide: 2994 dalton

    1 pmol = 2.994 ng

    1 ng   = 0.334 pmol

Proinsulin: 9395 dalton

    1 pmol = 9.395 ng

    1 ng   = 0.106 pmol

Clinical Syndromes Associated with Altered Insulin Receptor Function

Diminished Receptor Number

Obesity
Mild degree of NIDDM
Acanthosis nigricans type A
Leprechaunism
Insulinoma

Antireceptor Antibodies

Acanthosis nigricans type B
Ataxia-telangiectasia
(The two conditions are usually associated with insulin resistance. Occasionally antireceptor antibodies may mimic insulin action and produce hypoglycaemia.)

Increased Receptor Number

Anorexia nervosa

Causes of Insulin Resistance

Abnormal Beta Cell Secretory Product

Abnormal insulin molecule
Incomplete conversion of proinsulin to insulin

Circulating Insulin Antagonists

Elevated concentrations of counter-regulatory hormones (growth hormone, cortisol, glucagon, catecholamines)
Anti-insulin antibodies
Anti-insulin receptor antibodies
Amylin?

Target Tissue Defect

Insulin receptor defects
Post-receptor defects

Durability and Storage of Insulin

Seal unbroken, refrigerator:	Until expiration date
Seal broken, refrigerator:	Should not be stored in refrigerator
Seal unbroken, room temperature	1–2 months
Seal broken, room temperature:	1–2 months

For short periods of time insulin can be stored at temperatures higher than room temperature, but it should be placed in a refrigerator or in a cool place as soon as possible
Insulin, needles, syringes and insulin pen should always be carried in the hand luggage

Indications and Contraindications for Insulin Infuser Treatment

Indications

Poorly controlled diabetics in spite of correct conventional treatment with two to four insulin doses a day and a diet

Relative Contraindications

Physical handicaps
Psychosocial problems
Inability to recognize hypoglycaemic symptoms

Management of Practical Insulin Infuser Problems

Blood glucose <3 mmol/l:
Take a glass of juice or 5 g glucose. Check blood glucose 1 h later.

Extra snacks:
Take one to three units of regular insulin as a bolus, especially in case of intake of easily absorbable carbohydrates.

Delayed or early meals:
Take usual meal bolus.

Extra meal:
Take extra meal bolus.

Skipped meal:
Skip meal bolus.

Travel/holidays:
Always bring along fast- and intermediate-acting insulin and syringes for ordinary injection treatment in case of infuser failure, as well as extra batteries and catheters.

Sauna/swimming:
Take the infuser off.

Heat exposure:
Do not expose the infuser to direct sunlight or temperatures above 45°C (risk of insulin precipitation). Discard insulin which has been exposed to heat.

Cold exposure:
Always wear the infuser close to your body.

Infuser failure:
Call your doctor. Always carry insulin and syringes for conventional injection.

Air in cartridge and catheter:
Place cartridge and catheter upright with needle pointing upwards and press the button. Small air bubbles in cartridge/catheter do not cause trouble. 1 cm or less of air in the catheter is harmless.

Blocked catheter/blood in catheter:
Change catheter and site of infusion.

Smell of insulin:
Check needle and catheter as well as catheter and cartridge joint for leaks.

Tenderness at infusion site:
Change infusion site.

Inflammation at infusion site:
Change catheter, needle and infusion site. If the inflammation does not abate call doctor.

Sexual intercourse:
The infuser may be worn or may be taken off.

Infuser pause:
The infuser may be taken off for a maximum of 2 h just after a meal and a maximum of half an hour between meals. Take extra one to two units insulin bolus in case of a 2 h infusion pause.

Management of Insulin Infusion During Periods of Fever and Other Acute Episodes

Check blood glucose immediately before usual breakfast, lunch and dinner and at around 22.00 hours.

If food intake is normal give the usual meal boluses and, depending on blood glucose before the meal, an extra bolus (see table).

If the patient does not eat the usual meals, blood glucose should be checked as usual and insulin given (see table).

Blood glucose (mmol/l)	Fast-acting insulin (units, SC)
< 8	0
8– 9	1
9–11	2
11–13	3
> 13	4

If for unknown reasons blood glucose is > 13 mmol/l at bedtime, change catheter and check whether there are leaks or blockage in insulin infuser.

Diabetes in Childhood

Diagnosis

Thirst, polyuria, weight loss
Secondary enuresis
Abdominal pain
Hyperventilation
Recurrent carbuncles, perineal thrush

Laboratory Monitoring

Glycated haemoglobin (long-term control)
Fructosamine (short-term control)
Fingerstick glucose
First morning urine for glucose and ketones
Growth chart

Treatment Aims

Normoglycaemia using insulin
Eumetabolism
Maintenance of normal growth
Psychosocial equilibrium

Allergic Reactions to Insulin

Local Reactions

Immediate onset: Within 15 min – 2 h after injection.
Mediators: IgE antibodies.
Manifestations: Hard, indurated area at site of injection, brawny or erythematous rash. Occur after 1–4 weeks of prior exposure to intermediate- or long-acting insulin.
Treatment: Switch to monocomponent human insulin. Desensitization.

Delayed onset: 4 h or more after injection.
Mediators are IgG antibodies.
Lesions: As for immediate onset, develops over hours. Prior exposure generally 1–4 weeks after starting insulin therapy.
Treatment: As for immediate onset.

Systemic Reactions

Aetiological factors: History of intermittent insulin therapies, obesity, history of penicillin allergy, insulin resistance.
Mediators: IgE.
Manifestations: Generalized urticarial rash, angio-oedema, anaphylaxis, coexisting or antecedent local reactions.
Treatment: Adrenaline for immediate resuscitation, stop insulin, desensitization.

Desensitization Procedure[1]

Patient to stop insulin for at least 12–48 h. When necessary, give $NaHCO_3$ 1 g Q.I.D. to delay ketoacidosis.
Withhold all anti-allergic drugs.

---

[1] Galloway IA, Bressler R (1978) Insulin treatment in diabetes. Med Clin North Am 62:663–680.

Adrenaline (0.1–0.3 ml of 1:1000 solution) should be at hand. Decide to which animal species (beef or pork) desensitization is to be done.

Material
Desensitization materials are available in kits for different insulin types.

Dilution of regular insulin in the Eli Lilly insulin allergy desensitization kits

Bottle	Units/0.1 ml	Units/ml
A	1/1000	1/100
B	1/500	1/50
C	1/250	1/25
D	1/100	1/10
E	1/50	1/5
F	1/25	2/5
G	1/10	1
H	1/5	2
I	1/2	5
K	1	10

Method
The first ten desensitizing doses should be administered in 0.1 ml volumes every 30 min. The first three solutions (1/1000–1/250) are given intradermally. Subsequent dilutions are given SC.
If a positive reaction occurs, it is advisable to retreat by two dilutions.

Diabetic Ketoacidosis, Hyperosmolar Hyperglycaemic Non-ketotic Coma and Lactic Acidosis

Clinical Features of Diabetic Ketoacidosis (DKA)

Dehydration
Vomiting, abdominal pain, gastric dilatation
Overbreathing
Smell of ketones
Drowsiness of confusion
Coma (rare)
Hypothermia

Investigation and Treatment of Diabetic Ketoacidosis

	Initial	Over first 24 h
Physical examination	Level of consciousness Degree of dehydration tachypnoea, acetone foetor Cardiac status	Every 3–4 h

	Initial	Over first 24 h
Investigations	Urine output, urine glucose and ketones	Every hour
	Blood glucose, blood pressure, pulse, respiration rate, temperature, and body weight	Every 1–2 h
	ECG	p.r.n.
	Serum Na, K, CO_2, creatinine, haemoglobin, protein and pH	Every 4 h

NB! Enter all results on a flow sheet.

Further investigations	Find cause of DKA
	History and physical examination
	Blood and urine culture and sensitivity
	Chest X-ray, lumbar puncture, white blood cell and differential blood count
Additional treatment if necessary	Antibiotics
	Nasogastric aspiration if there is any degree of impaired consciousness or the patient is vomiting. Aspirate hourly
	Urinary catheter if there is no spontaneous urine output after 1 h or if the patient is too ill to provide an accurate urine output
	Transfer to intensive case unit in case of respiratory problems, shock, arrhythmia or severe potassium disturbances
	IV fluid and insulin should "hot" be continued until the patient is drinking and eating without vomiting

Treatment of Diabetic Ketoacidosis in Adults (Over 15 Years)

	STATIM	0–1 h	2 h	3 h
Fast-acting insulin IV	10 units	5 units/h	5 units/h	5 units/h
0.9% NaCl		1500 ml	500 ml	125 ml
KCl (mmol/h)				
K < 3:	39	39	39	39
3–4:	26	26	26	26
4–5:	13	13	13	13
> 5:	0	0	0	0

Bicarbonate
  If CO_2 < 10 mmol/l
  or pH < 7.10
	75–100 mmol over 45 min.
	Repeat until pH > 7.0
	Add 10–20 mmol KCl			

When blood glucose has fallen to < 14 mmol/l, infuse glucose 5% or 0.9% NaCl plus 5% glucose.

Once the patient is able to eat and drink and the acidosis has disappreared (CO_2 > 22 mmol/l), proceed with SC fast-acting insulin before the meal. Stop IV insulin and glucose 20–30 min after SC injection.

Treatment of Diabetic Ketoacidosis in Children (Under 15 Years)

	STATIM	0–1 h	2 h	3 h
Fast-acting insulin IV (units/kg)	0.3	0.1	0.1	0.1
0.9% NaCl (ml/kg)	25	25	10	5
KCl (mmol/kg · h)				
K < 3:	0.6	0.6	0.6	0.6
3–4:	0.4	0.4	0.4	0.4
4–5:	0.3	0.3	0.3	0.3
5–6:	0.2	0.2	0.2	0.2
> 6:	Stop			
Bicarbonate If CO_2 < 10 mmol/l or pH < 7.10	Amount (mmol): [12 − CO_2 (mmol/l) × body weight (kg)] − 0.4. Half amount in $\frac{1}{2}$ h and rest in 1–2 h. Repeat until pH > 7.0. Extra K 0.2 mmol/kg over 3 h			

When blood glucose has fallen to < 14 mmol/l, and once the child is able to eat and drink, continue infusion and IV insulin until next meal; then give SC fast-acting insulin 20 min before the meal. Stop IV fluid and insulin 20–30 min after SC insulin.

Calculation of Potassium Deficit, Plasma Osmolarity, pH and Anion Gap

Potassium Deficit

Normal $-$ actual serum K (mmol/l) $\times$ body weight (kg) = K deficit

Plasma Osmolarity

$2 \times$ Na (mmol/l) + blood glucose (mmol/l) + serum urea (mmol/l)
= Osmolarity (mosmol/kg) (reference range 276–295)

pH

$$pH = pK + \log \frac{(HCO_3)}{(H_2CO_3)} \quad \text{or}$$

$$pH = 6.1 + \log \frac{(HCO_3)}{0.03 \times PaCO_2} \quad \text{(Henderson-Hasselbalch equation)}$$

Anion gap

Na $-$ [(HCO$_3$) + Cl] = 8–12 mmol/l (normal)

If anion gap $>$ 12 mmol/l: accumulation of acetoacetic acid, β-hydroxybutyrate, lactic acid, phosphate and sulphate is likely

Corrected Sodium

For each 5.6 mmol/l increment in plasma glucose above the normal levels, the serum sodium concentration can be expected to be decreased by 1.6 mmol/l

In order to estimate the "corrected" sodium concentration – the sodium concentration if the osmotic effect of glucose were removed – one may use the following equation:

Corrected Na (mmol/l)

$$= \text{Measured Na (mmol/l)} + \frac{\text{Plasma glucose (mmol/l)} - 5.6}{3.4}$$

Hazards of Severe Acidaemia and Alkali Therapy

Acidaemia (pH < 7)

Negative inotropic effect
Peripheral vasodilatation
Hypotension
Cerebral depression
Insulin resistance

Alkali therapy

Hypokalaemia
Impaired oxyhaemoglobin disssociation
Paradoxical fall in pH in cerebrospinal fluid
Rebound alkalosis
Sodium overload

Biochemical Deficits in Severe Diabetic Ketoacidosis

Element	Quantity
Water	5–6 l
Sodium	500 mmol/l
Chloride	350 mmol/l
Potassium	300–1000 mmol/l
Magnesium	10–25 mmol/l
Phosphate	25–50 mmol/l

Treatment of Hyperosmolar Hyperglycaemic Non-ketotic Coma (HHNC)

Immediate	Subsequent
0.9% NaCl, 1 l/h; replace Na deficit in 4–6 h (500 mmol/l)	When blood pressure stable, urine output adequate, change to 0.45% NaCl, 250–500 ml/h
	When blood glucose < 14 mmol/l add 5% glucose to IV fluid Replace H_2O deficit over 12–24 h (5–10 l)
If serum K high, begin KCl 20 mmol/l after urine output established	Adjust dose of KCl by serial serum K
If serum K normal or low, begin KCl 20 mmol/l immediately; measure K hourly	
Fast-acting insulin 0.05–0.10 units/kg/h IV	Decrease infusion rate to 1–3 units/h; when eating, switch to SC insulin;
Monitor blood glucose hourly	Monitor glucose and electrolytes every 4 h

Comparison of Hyperosmolar Hyperglycaemic Non-ketotic Coma (HHNC) and Diabetic Ketoacidosis (DKA)[1]

Clinical picture	HHNC	DKA
General	More dehydrated Not acidotic Frequently coma No hyperventilation	Less dehydrated More acidotic Rarely coma Hyperventilation
Age	Usually elderly	Younger patients
Type	NIDDM	IDDM
Previous history of diabetes	In only 50%	Almost always
Prodromes	Several days	Less than 1 day
Neurological symptoms and signs	Very common	Rare
Underlying renal or cardiovascular disease	About 85%	About 15%

Laboratory findings
  Blood glucose
    (mmol/l)
	>44	Usually <44

Serum Na	N, elevated, low	Usually low
Serum K	N or elevated	Elevated, N, low
Serum CO_2 (mmol/l)	>16	<10
Anion gap (mmol/l)	10–12	>12
Blood pH	N	<7.35

---

[1] Kosac GP, Rolla AR (1982) Diabetic comas. In: Kozak GP (ed) Clinical diabetes mellitus. Saunders, Philadelphia, p. 132.

Clinical picture	HHNC	DKA
Serum osmolarity (mosmol/l)	> 350	<350
Serum BUN	higher than DKA	lower than HHNC
FFA (mmol/l)	<1	>1.5
Complications		
Thrombosis	Frequent	Rare
Mortality (%)	20–50	1–10

N, normal, BUN, blood urea nitrogen; FFA, free fatty acids

Lactic Acidosis

Diagnostic criteria	pH <7.35, blood lactate >5–6 mmol/l
Aetiology	Biguanides
	Tissue hypoxia (volume contraction, micro- and macrovascular disease)
	Decreased haemoglobin affinity for O_2 due to decreased 2,3-diphosphoglycerate
	Increased blood viscosity
	Insulin lack leads to decreased pyruvate de-hydrogenase activity
Symptoms	Tachypnoea, dehydration, abdominal pain, drowsiness and coma

Treatment	Rehydration
	Replace insulin lack
	Treat underlying ailments (infection, cardiac failure).
	Iudicious use of bicarbonate infusion when indicated in severe cases (pH <7.2, HCO_3 <10–12 mmol/l)
	Dialysis for severe cases with co-existing renal failure or severe congestive heart failure
Hazards of alkali therapy	Leftward shift of O_2 dissociation curve
	Reduction of tissue oxygenation in low output states
	Hyperosmolar state or cardiac failure (high Na load)
	Rebound alkalosis from metabolism of lactate to HCO_3
	Hypokalaemia and hypercalcaemia
	Paradoxical CSF acidosis
	Aggravation of acidaemia (increased CO_2 production)
	Contentious evidence of real benefit on survival
	Myocardial depression (rapid intramyocardial cellular acidosis)
	Carbicarb (equimolar solution of $NaHCO_3$ plus Na_2CO_3 may be safer than HCO_3 alone)

Commonly Used Solutions for Parenteral Infusion

	Na	K	Ca	NH$_4$	Cl	CO$_2$[a]	Glucose (g/l)	(kJ)	(mosmol/l)
	(mEq/l)								
5% glucose							50	795	280
10% glucose							100	1590	560
0.9% NaCl	155				155				310
5% NaCl	861				861				1722
Ringer's solution	147	4	4		155				310
Ringer's lactate	130	4	3		109	28			274
Darrow's solution	121	35			103	53			312
KCl 0.2% in 5% glucose		27			27		50	190	334
KCl 0.3% in 5% glucose		40			40		50	190	360
Ammonium chloride 0.9%				170	170				340
Na lactate 1,4%	153					153			306
Na bicarbonate 1,7%	167				167				334

[a] Bicarbonate equivalent may be lactate, acetate, gluconate or citrate, or combinations of these. A variety of modifications of multiple electrolyte solutions are commercially available.

Acute Diabetic Emergencies

Comas
    Hypoglycaemia
    Ketoacidotic
    Hyperosmolar hyperglycaemic non-ketotic (HHNC)
    Lactic acidosis
    Uraemia
    Non-diabetic comas
Infection
Myocardial infarction
Stroke
Emergency surgery

Hypoglycaemia

Aetiology

Endogenous Hypoglycaemia

Hyperinsulinaemia (insulinoma, nesidioblastosis, insulin antibodies)
Endocrinopathy (adrenal, pituitary, glucagon deficiencies)
Reactive (post-gastrectomy)
Liver disease
Paraneoplastic (hepatoma, mesenchymal tumour, lymphoma etc.)
Septicaemic states
Cardiac failure
Uraemia
Insulin receptor antibodies (rare)

Exogenous Hypoglycaemia

Diabetes related:
IDDM patient on insulin
  Skipped meals, ritual fasting, slimming, unaccustomed exercise,
wrong dose, dialysis, brittle diabetes, change in insulin requirement,
defective counter-regulation
Surreptitious use of antidiabetic medication:
  Insulin (plasma C peptide low)
  Oral antidiabetic drugs
  Other drugs (salicylates, propranolol, perhexiline, propoxyphene,
  p-aminosalicylic acid (PAS), acetaminophen, colchicine, disopy-
  ramide, monoamine oxidase (MAO) inhibitors

Differential Diagnosis of Hypoglycaemia with Hyperinsulinaemia

	Blood glucose	Fasting insulin (μU/ml)	C peptide	Other
Insulinoma	Low	10–50	High	Localize tumour
Surreptitious insulin	Low	$>$ 50	Low	Insulin antibodies
Sulphonylurea	Low	10–50	High	Drug assay
Auto-immune	Low	$>$200	Low	Insulin antibodies

Symptoms

Blood glucose level (mmol/l)	Symptoms
4	Asymptomatic
3–3.5	Decreased attention, impaired fine motor skills and reaction time
2–3	Palpitations, arrhythmia, anxiety, pallor, sweating, hunger, drowsiness, mental deterioration, slowing of EEG, lethargy etc.
$<$2	Frank coma
1–2	Seizures, irreversible brain damage, death

Causes of Hypoglycaemia in Insulin-Dependent Diabetes Mellitus

Insulin	Inappropriate insulin regimes
	Day-to-day variability in absorption
	Insulin antibodies
	Inappropriate site rotation
	Factitious hypoglycaemia
	Renal failure
Food	Delayed intake
	Decreased intake
Exercise	Increased energy requirements
	Increased insulin absorption
Other	Impaired counter-regulation and "unawareness"
	Liver disease
	Hypoendocrine disorders
	Alcohol
	Drugs (salicylates, pentamidine, perhexiline, propranolol, propoxyphene, PAS, acetaminophen, colchicine, disopyramide, MAO inhibitors)

Approach to Patients

History

Diabetes, type and dose of treatment
Other drugs
Other medical conditions
Time of onset of symptoms in relation to drugs and meals
Antecedent events (exercise, fasting, illness etc.)

Physical Examination

Autonomic signs
Neuroglycopenic signs
General systemic examination

Document hypoglycaemia and note abatement of associated features after acute normalization of blood glucose (Whipple's triad).

If mechanism for hypoglycaemia is obvious, no further diagnostic evaluation is necessary; continue restitutive measures.

Proceed to investigations if mechanism of hypoglycaemia is not obvious.

Investigations

Measure plasma glucose after overnight fast.

If post-absorptive hypoglycaemia is documented proceed to:
Plasma insulin and C peptide determination, screen blood or urine for sulphonylurea and metabolites, check blood alcohol level.

If unresolved proceed to:
Insulin antibody titres, serum tumour markers, e.g. carcinoembryonic antigen (CEA), α-fetoprotein, insulin-like growth factors, β-human chorionic gonadotropin (βhCG), and radiological search for tumour.

If still unresolved:
Screen for deficiency of counter-regulation: basal plasma catecholamins, glucagon, cortisol, growth hormone; dynamic testing for hormone deficiencies.

Treatment

If blood glucose is <3 mmol/l and the patient is able to drink, give a glass of juice, 10 g glucose or about 20 g cane sugar orally.

If the patient is unconscious inject immediately 50 ml 50% glucose IV. Continue with IV infusion of 5% glucose.

If immediate access to peripheral vein is impossible, inject 1 mg glucagon IM.

If the patient is still unconscious 30 min after normalization of blood glucose, the reason might be incipient cerebral oedema. Rule out other causes of unconsciousness. Bolus injection of dexamethasone 12 mg IV is given, followed by mannitol 40 g IV in the course of 20 min.

Adverse Effects

Behavioural change, intellectual impairment
Unconsciousness
Accidents
Myocardial infarction
Hemiparesis
Mental deterioration
Locked-in syndrome
Vegetative state

Surgery in Diabetic Patients

Management of Adult Diabetic Patients (over 12 Years) During Surgery

Insulin-Dependent Diabetic Patients

Minor Surgery
If first on morning list:
- No morning insulin.
- Check blood glucose pre-op: 6–13 mmol/l – proceed with operation. >13 mmol/l – give insulin and glucose as for major surgery. <6 mmol/l – set up 5% glucose drip.
- Monitor blood glucose every 2 h as well as immediately pre- and post-op.
- By lunch-time patient should be able to eat and drink, so give half morning insulin as fast-acting (soluble) insulin with lunch.
- Give normal evening insulin.

If procedure is later in day:
- Give half the patient's normal morning insulin as fast-acting with a light breakfast (finishing 4–6 h before procedure).
- Check blood glucose pre- and post-op and proceed as above, depending on result.
- Monitor blood glucose every 2 h
- The patient should be able to eat and drink by supper-time, when he or she can have the normal insulin.

Major Surgery
- The patient should be admitted to hospital not later than the morning before the day of surgery.
- Check blood glucose at 11.00, 17.00 and 20.00 hours on day of admission, and also at 07.00 on the day of surgery.
- If operation before 12.00 hours, omit breakfast and morning insulin. If after, give light breakfast and half normal insulin as fast-acting (soluble).
- Check urine for glucose and ketones.
- Check serum electrolytes (Na, K, creatinine, and if needed CO_2).
- ECG.

Basic pre-surgery requirements:
- Blood glucose 4–14 mmol/l
- No ketoacidosis
- Normohydration
- No acute ECG changes

Pre-operatively:
- Consult internist if above requirements are not fulfilled.
- Surgery should be performed early in the morning.
- Premedication required.
- It should be noted in the surgical record that the patient is a diabetic.

Day of surgery:
- STATIM blood glucose, fasting, at 07.00 hours.
- Give 10% glucose plus 10 mEq KCl/l. Infusion rate 80–120 ml/h.
- Give IV insulin via a syringe pump containing 50 units fast-acting (soluble) insulin in 50 ml 0.9% NaCl, i.e. 1 unit/ml. Start at 2 units/h.
- Check blood glucose every hour and alter insulin infusion rate according to sliding scale:

Blood glucose (mmol/l)	Insulin infusion (units/h)
< 4	$\frac{1}{2}$ (inform doctor)
4–7	1
7–11	2
11–17	4
> 17	6

– Check blood glucose post-op and then every 2 h

Post-operatively:
– Continue IV infusion and check blood glucose and electrolytes, including bicarbonate, immediately after surgery.
– Check blood glucose approximately every 4–6 h until the patient can eat and drink.
– Give fast-acting insulin (about $\frac{1}{3}$ of previous total daily dose) 20 min before the meal. Stop IV insulin and glucose 30–60 min after SC injection.

Non-Insulin-Dependent Diabetic Patients

Minor Surgery
Patients treated with diet:
– Avoid glucose-containing solutions.
– Check blood glucose pre- and post-op and 6 h later.
– Where normal food intake is expected to be resumed during the day of operation: No special treatment.

Well-controlled patients treated with oral antidiabetic drugs:
– If possible stop biguanide and long-acting sulphonylurea 48 h before.
– Where normal food intake is expected to be resumed during the day of operation the tablet can be administered with the first meal after the operation.
– Check blood glucose pre- and post-op and every 4 h until recovery.

Major Surgery or Poorly Controlled Patients
- Convert to SC fast-acting insulin Q.I.D. for at least 48 h pre- and post-op and then manage as IDDM peri-op.

Management of Diabetic Children (Under 12 Years) During Surgery

General Guideline

The paediatrician should be informed about children admitted for surgery.

Minor Surgery

- Admit on the day of surgery.
- The child should be placed first on the operating list.
- Check pre-op blood glucose and urine for ketones.
- Check blood glucose post-op and again at 2 h.

For morning lists:
- The child's parents should have been instructed to reduce the previous night's long-acting insulin by half.
- Omit the morning insulin.
- The child should be awake and able to drink and eat by lunch-time.
- Give fast-acting (soluble) insulin pre-lunch – about 50% of the normal morning insulin dose.
- Give normal evening dose.

For afternoon lists:
- Give half normal morning insulin and early breakfast.
- The child should be awake and able to eat and drink by supper-time.
- Give normal insulin at supper.

Major Surgery

- For routine major surgery, admit the day before.
- Check urea and electrolytes and blood glucose.
- Check urine for ketones.
- Check pre-meal and bedtime blood glucose.
- Reduce evening long-acting insulin by half, if well controlled
- Omit normal SC insulin on morning of the operation.
- Set up a drip of 10% glucose and 0.45% NaCl with 10 mmol KCl per 500 ml of fluid:

Child's weight (kg)	Fluid (ml/kg · 24 h)
10	100
18	80
30	60
50	50

- Insulin should be given IV using an insulin pump at a rate determined by the blood glucose as follows:

Blood glucose (mmol/l)	Insulin infusion rate (units/kg · h)
>10	0.1
5–10	0.05
<5	0.03

- Check blood glucose every 2 h.
- If blood glucose runs high (>10 mmol/l) for 4 h or more, increase the pump rate to 0.15 units/kg · h, but only after checking that the pump is working and connected to a functioning IV line.
- Continue IV regimen until child is able to eat and drink normally.
- Check urea and electrolytes after the operation and then if infusion is prolonged (>12 h) do twice daily.
- Once child is able to eat and drink, continue infusion and IV insulin until next meal, then give SC insulin 20 min before the meal, either previous normal dose if breakfast or supper, or 30% of total daily dose as fast-acting if lunch. Stop IV fluids and insulin 20–30 min after the SC insulin.

Pregnancy in Diabetic Patients

White's Classification (Slightly Modified) of Maternal and Neonatal Risk

Category	Age at diagnosis (years)		Duration of diabetes (years)	Background retinopathy
A	NIDDM			
B	>20	and	<10	0
C	10–19	or	10–19	0
D	<10	or	>20	+
F	Nephropathy and/or proliferative retinopathy			

Maternal and Neonatal Risks Increase from A to F.

Evaluation of the Foetoplacental Unit During Pregnancy

System	Investigations	Time
Neural tube	α-foetoprotein in amniotic fluid Amniocentesis	Week 16
Foetal weight	Biparietal diameter Abdominal volume Length of femur Ultrasound	Week 30 and 36
Foetal heartbeat	Cardiotocography	Week 36 to birth, 2–4 times/week
Placental function	Plasma human placental lactogen	If obstetrically indicated
Foetoplacental unity	Urinary oestriol	If obstetrically indicated

Congenital Malformations in Infants of Diabetic Mothers

Caudal regression
Spina bifida, hydrocephalus and other CNS defects
Anencephaly

Transposition of great vessels
Ventricular septal defect
Atrial septal defect

Anal/rectal atresia

Renal agenesis
Cystic kidney
Double ureter
Situs inversus viscerum

Clinical Disorders in Infants of Diabetic Mothers

Macrosomia
Hypoglycaemia
Hypocalcaemia
Respiratory distress syndrome
Polycythaemia
Hyperviscocity
Hyperbilirubinaemia
Renal vein thrombosis
Persistence of foetal circulation
Cardiomyopathy
Congenital anomalies

Prognostically Bad Signs During Pregnancy

Clinical pyelonephritis
Pre-coma or severe ketoacidosis
Toxaemia
Non-compliance

Recommendations for Screening
for Gestational Diabetes Mellitus

Routine urine analysis for glucose at all visits. If any tests are positive a postprandial blood glucose screening is indicated.

At 24–28 weeks, a postprandial blood glucose screening test for all women not previously identified as having glucose intolerance.

For high-risk patients, a post-prandial blood glucose screening test at 12–18 weeks, 26 weeks and 32 weeks if previous tests are negative or oral glucose tolerance tests are negative.

If any of the plasma glucose screening tests are positive an oral glucose tolerance test is indicated

High-Risk Patients

Previous gestational diabetes
Family history of diabetes
Obesity
Previous high-birth-weight infants
Obstetric history of stillbirth, prematurity or polyhydramnios
Essential or pregnancy-induced hypertension
Renal glycosuria

Non-Insulin-Dependent Diabetes Mellitus

Risk Factors

Genetic (>90% concordance among monozygotic twins)
Obesity
Age
Sedentary life-style
Dietary factors
Stress
Urbanization
Acculturation
Social factors

Treatment Flow Scheme

AIM: No glycosuria, postprandial blood glucose <10 mmol/l, normal glycosylated haemoglobin.

Non-obese	Obese
Weight-maintaining diabetes diet	Weight-reducing diabetes diet
If no effect: Weight-maintaining diet + sulphonylurea	If no effect: Weight-reducing diet + sulphonylurea or metformin
If no effect: Weight-maintaining diet + insulin	If no effect: Weight-reducing diet + insulin

Clinical Pharmacology of Oral Antidiabetic Drugs

Drug	Maximum plasma concentration (h)	Plasma half-life (h)	Plasma albumin binding	Metabolism	Metabolites in urine	Duration of action (h)	Usual 24-h dose (mg)
Tolbutamide	3–6	5–8	Ionic	Liver	Inactive	6–12	500 b.i.d.–t.i.d.
Chlorpropamide	2–4	36	–	Liver	Active?	36	125–250 q.d.
Tolazamide	4–8	8	–	Liver	3 active 3 slightly active	24	100–500 q.d.
Glibenclamide	1–2	4–6	Non-ionic	Liver	Inactive	24	1.75–3.5 q.d. to b.i.d.
Glipizide	1	2–4	–	Liver	Inactive	24	2.5–7.0 b.i.d.
Glibornuride	2–4	8	–	Liver	Inactive	8–10	12.5–50 t.i.d.
Gliclazide	3–7	6–14	–	Liver	Inactive	12	40–80 q.d. to b.i.d.
Metformin	2	3	None	None	Secreted unchanged	24	500 t.i.d. or 850 b.i.d.

Side-Effects of Sulphonylureas and Biguanides

Sulphonylureas

Hypoglycaemia
Dyspepsia
Exanthema
Alcohol-Antabuse reaction
Liver-bone marrow toxicity (rare)

Biguanides

Malaise
Dyspepsia, anorexia, nausea, diarrhoea
Lactic acidosis (rare with metformin)
Vitamin 12 and folate deficiency
Liver and kidney toxicity

Interactions of Sulphonylureas

Substances Antagonizing Sulphonylurea Actions

Impair insulin release or action
    Thiazides and furosemide
    Phenytoin
    Beta-blockers
    Diazoxide
    Corticosteroids
    Oestrogens
    Isoniazid
    Indomethacin
    Nicotinic acid

Shorten sulphonylurea half-life via enzyme induction
   Alcohol
   Rifampin

Mechanism unclear
   Phenothiazines
   Acetazolamide

Substances Potentiating Sulphonylurea Actions and Causing Profound Hypoglycaemia

Displacement of sulphonylurea from plasma protein binding sites
   Sulphonamides
   Salicylates
   Pyrazolone derivatives (phenylbutazone, sulphinpyrazone, oxyphenbutazone)
   Clofibrate
   Halofenate

Prolong sulphonylurea half-life via competition for enzyme
   Bishydroxycoumarin (dicumarol)
   Chloramphenicol
   Pyrazolone derivatives
   Monoamine oxidase inhibitors
   Sulphaphenazole

Decrease urinary excretion of sulphonylureas and their metabolites
   Probenecid
   Salicylates
   Pyrazolone derivatives
   Sulphonamides
   Allopurinol

Enhance sulphonylurea's hypoglycaemic effect
  Salicylates
  Guanethidine
  Beta-blockers
  Monoamine oxidase inhibitors
  Alcohol

Contraindications for Sulphonylurea Treatment

IDDM or pancreatic diabetes
Pregnancy
Surgery
Severe infections
History of severe adverse reaction to sulphonylurea
Patients with severe liver or kidney disease (risk of hypoglycaemia)

Mechanism of Action of Sulphonylureas

Pancreatic
Improved insulin secretion
Reduced glucagon secretion

Extrapancreatic
Improved tissue sensitivity to insulin
  Direct
    Increased receptor binding
    Improved postbinding action
  Indirect
    Reduced hyperglycaemia
    Decreased plasma free fatty acids
Reduced hepatic insulin extraction

Diabetic Foot Syndrome

Classification of Foot Ulcers

Grade	Lesion
1	Superficial
2	Deep
3	Abscess/osteomyelitis
4	Minor gangrene
5	Major gangrene

Other Foot Problems

Charcot Joint

Swollen, erythematous, inflamed foot
Radiographic evidence of bone lesion/fracture
Predilection for metatarsal joints
Bone scan shows increased tracer uptake
Treatment supportive

Neuropathic Oedema

Swelling of feet and lower legs associated with severe neuropathy
Underlying vasomotor abnormality and arteriovenous shunting in distal limbs
Ephedrine 30 mg PO t.i.d. sometimes useful

Prevention of Foot Ulcers

Wash and inspect feet daily
Lubricate feet with talc or lanolin
Regular chiropodic visits
Adaptive shoes to reduce foot pressure
Strict control of diabetes

Role of Surgery in Foot Ulcers

Debridement of devitalized areas
Vascular surgery in selected cases
Ray amputation of toe(s) with underlying bone destruction
More extensive amputation of gangrenous limbs
Early joint care with orthopaedic surgeon preferable

Clinical Characteristics of Ischaemic and Neuropathic Foot Ulcers

	Ischaemic	Neuropathic
Localization	Distally on toes On dorsal foot On crus as fat necrosis	On tips of toes Over metatarsal capitulum Where skin is under pressure
Appearance	Skin is cool No pulse No hair Pain	Normal skin temperature Normal pulse Normal hair No pain
Treatment	Keep dry Immobilize	Chloramine dressing Remove callosities Relieve pressure with therapeutic shoes
Examinations	Measure arterial pressure	Measure arterial pressure

Treatment of Infected Foot Ulcers and Osteitis

Foot Ulcers

Unclean ulcers: Culture after rinsing with saline. Change chloramine dressing (0.1%) morning and noon until culture result is available. In the evening use either chloramine or 0.1% chlorhexidine to keep the ulcer moist until next morning.

In case of infection with *Pseudomonas aeruginosa:* Change from chloramine to aluminium acetate (sol. aluminii subacetatis 0.8%). If no *Pseudomonas* infection: Continue with chloramine or chlorhexidine.

Osteitis

In case of active osteitis *without* ulcer: Do blood culture three times and start treatment with penicillin injections 2 g t.i.d. until erythrocyte sedimentation rate (ESR) falls. Then, dicloxacillin 1 g PO t.i.d. for 2–3 weeks.

In case of osteitis *with* ulcer: Culture and until the result of this is available, treat as for osteitis without ulcer. If test result makes changes necessary consult microbiologist.

Indications for Peripheral Vascular Surgery

Noctural pain
Rest pain
Foot ulcers unresponsive to treatment
Infection unresponsive to treatment
Incipient gangrene
Severe disabling intermittent claudication

Chance of Healing (%) after Amputation in Relation to Pre-operative Distal Blood Pressure and Skin Perfusion Pressure[1]

	Pressure (mmHg)		
	<20	21–30	>30
Toe (distal BP pressure)	Very low	–	High
Ankle (distal BP pressure)	0	38	57
Crus (skin perfusion)	25	67	94
Thigh (skin perfusion)	–	9[a]	75

[a] Figure applied for pressure <30 mmHg.

Diabetic Macrovascular Disease Risk Factors

Treatable

Smoking
Hypertension
Hypercholesterolaemia
Hypertriglyceridaemia
Hyperglycaemia

---

[1] From PE Holstein (1985) Skin perfusion pressure measured by radioisotope washout for predicting wound healing in lower limb amputation for arterial occlusive disease (thesis). Acta Orthop Scand (Suppl 213).

Not Treatable

Genetic
Age
Diabetic phenotype
Duration of diabetes

Diabetic Nephropathy

Some Definitions

Normoalbuminuria <30 mg/24 h
Microalbuminuria 30–250 mg/24 h (incipient nephropathy)
Macroalbuminuria >250 mg/24 h (clinical nephropathy)

Follow-Up of Patients

Check for microalbuminuria once a year in diabetic patients with diabetes of more than 5 years' duration

Diabetic Patients with Microalbuminuria

Measure urinary albumin excretion quantitatively once a year
Aim at normoglycaemia
Measure blood pressure every 3 months
Treat rise in blood pressure ($>140/90$ mm Hg)

Diabetic Patients with Intermittent Macroalbuminuria

Exclude urinary tract infection
Measure serum creatinine and blood pressure every 3 months
Do ECG and ophthalmoscopy

Diabetic Patients with Persistent Macroalbuminuria

As for "intermittent macroalbuminuria"
Refer to nephrology unit when plasma creatinine is 300 μmol/l
Consider dialysis or renal transplant when glomerular filtration rate is
15 ml/min

Treatment of Urinary Tract Infection

Examine urine for leucocytes, haematuria and bacteriuria (culture plus
sensitivity).

If there are symptoms, start antibiotic treatment:
– Patients who *have not* had urinary tract infection in the last year:
   sulphamethizole 1 g + 1 g 3 h later PO.
– Patients who *have had* urinary tract infection two to three times in
   the last year: ampicillin 500 mg t.i.d. PO for 3 days.
– Patients with *several episodes* of urinary tract infection: Sulfame-
   thoxazole 400 mg + trimethoprim 80 mg PO at bedtime for 1 month
   or even longer depending on the urine culture.

If there are no symptoms, consider treatment in case of significant
bacteriuria. Pyuria without symptoms need not be treated. In case of
sterile pyuria check for tuberculosis.

Indications for Dialysis or Kidney Transplantation

Absolute

Serum creatinine >700 μmol/l
Creatinine clearance <5 ml/min
Uraemic gastritis, colitis, pericarditis, seizures
Unremitting weight loss, decline in muscle mass

Relative

Serum creatinine 350–700 μmol/l
Failure to thrive, lethargy
Unresponsive oedema
Progressive retinopathy/neuropathy
Nausea, bloating, abdominal discomfort

Available Uraemic Therapies

Haemodialysis
Haemofiltration
Peritoneal dialysis (intermittent/continuous)
Renal transplantation (living/cadaver donor)

Preparing Diabetics for Uraemic Therapy

Visit to haemodialysis and peritoneal dialysis units
Meet transplant patient
Discussion with transplant surgeon
Family conference to consider living donor
Creation of vascular access for haemodialysis
Inventory and tissue-type potential kidney donors
Identify patients specific primary physician

Conditions Affecting the Kidney in Diabetes

Urinary tract infections
Contrast media-induced nephropathy
Atonic bladder/hydronephrosis
Nephrosclerosis
Atherosclerosis
Diffuse and/or nodular intercapillary glomerulosclerosis

Diabetic Neuropathy

Classification

Somatic Peripheral Neuropathy

Deep tendon areflexia
Decreased vibratory perception
Hypaesthesia
Dysaesthesia
Paraesthesia

Autonomic Neuropathy

Diarrhoea
Gastroparesis
Diabetic enteropathy/malabsorption
Postural hypotension
Cardiovascular dysfunction
Gustatory sweating/anhidrosis
Neurogenic bladder
Impotence
Retrograde ejaculation
Atonic pupil
Vasomotor instability

Asymmetric Neuropathies

Extraocular muscle palsies
Other mononeuropathies
Diabetic amyotrophy

Test for Autonomic Neuropathy

Parasympathetic

Heart rate response to Valsalva manoeuvre
Beat-to-beat variation during breathing
Immediate heart rate response to standing

Sympathetic

Blood pressure response to standing
Blood pressure response to sustained handgrip

Methods

Heart rate response to Valsalva manoeuvre:
– Patient blows into manometer and holds breath at 40 mm Hg for 15 s
– Continuous ECG: Repeat 3 times after 1 min rest
– Risky in patients with proliferative retinopathy
– *Result:* Largest R-R interval after Valsalva manoeuvre divided by shortest R-R interval during manoeuvre

Immediate heart rate response to standing:
- Patient connected to ECG lying down
- Patient abruptly stands up
- Measure shortest R-R interval around the 15th beat and largest interval around 30th beat on standing
- *Result:* Calculate the 30:15 ratio

Beat-to-beat variation during breathing:
- Patient rests on couch for 5 min connected to ECG
- Switch on ECG
- Patient breathes deeply and holds breath for 5 s, then exhales quickly, stopping for 5 s
- Repeat procedure five times
- Press test button on ECG at onset of each inspiration
- *Result:* Maximum pulse rate minus minimum pulse rate for inspiration and expiration. Calculate mean

Sustained handgrip:
- Use handgrip dynamometer and find patient's maximum voluntary contraction
- Patient maintains grip at one-third maximum for 5 min
- Check blood pressure three times before and at 1- min intervals during handgrip
- *Result:* Highest diastolic blood pressure during grip minus mean basal diastolic blood pressure

Interpretation[1]

	Normal	Border-line	Abnormal
Heart rate ration during and after Valsalva manoeuvre	> 1.21	1.11–1.20	< 1.10
R-R variation on deep breathing (max. minus min.)	>15/min	11–14	<10
Immediate heart rate on standing (30:15 ratio)	> 1.04	1.01– 1.03	< 1.00
Blood pressure response to standing (systolic drop)	<10	11–29	>30
Blood pressure response to handgrip	>16	11–15	<10

Treatment Protocol for Pain Relief[2]

Neuropathic pain confirmed:
- Simple analgesic (aspirin, paracetamol, mefenamic acid)

Simple analgesic fails:
- Imipramine 50 mg nocte
- Increase stepwise to 150 mg nocte as required

[1] Ewing DJ, Clarke BF (1982) Diagnosis and management of diabetic autonomic neuropathy. Br Med J 285:916–918.
[2] Young RJ, Clarke BF (1985) Pain relief in diabetic neuropathy: the effectiveness of imipramine and related drugs. Diabetic Med 2:363–366.

Intolerant of imipramine (dry mouth, dizziness, hesitancy):
– Mianserin 30 mg nocte
– Increase stepwise to 90 mg nocte as required

Imipramine tolerated but insufficient:
– Substitute amitriptyline 50–150 mg nocte ± chlorpromazine
   50–100 mg per day or fluphenazine 1–6 mg per day

If severe "restless legs" or above failed:
– Clonazepam 0.5–3 mg

Maximum response in less than 6 months
– Try to withdraw treatment

Diabetic Eye Disease

Occular Manifestation of Diabetes

Retina

Diabetic retinopathy
Vein occlusion
Lipaemia retinalis

Vitreous

Sequelae of diabetic retinopathy
Asteroid hyalosis

Lens

Cataract
Transient opacifications
Fluctuations in refraction

Pupil

Sluggish response
Small pupil
Argyl-Robertson pupil
Neuropathy with pupillary involvement

Optic Nerve

Optic atrophy
Optic neuropathy
DIDMOAD (diabetes insipidus, diabetes mellitus, optic atrophy, deafness)

Ciliary Body

Weakness of accommodation
Basement membrane thickening

Iris

Vacuolation
Pigment dispersion
Ectropion uveae

Cornea

Wrinkles
Pigmentation
Decreased sensitivity

Nerves, Extraocular Muscles

Neuropathy

Ocular Appendages

Blepharitis, xanthelasma
Abnormalities of conjunctival vasculature

Orbit

Cellulitis, mucormycosis

Diabetic Retinopathy

Background

Phlebopathy
Microaneurysms
Exudates (hard/soft)
Haemorrhages

Maculopathy

Haemorrhages, exudates, and oedema in the macular region

Pre-proliferative

Large, deep, round haemorrhages, soft exudates, phlebopathy, venous reduplication, obliterated small arterioles

Proliferative

Intraretinal microvascular abnormalities (IRMA), proliferations, corpus vitreum haemorrhages, fibrosis, retinal detachment, haemorrhagic glaucoma

Follow-Up of Patients with Diabetic Retinopathy

Ophthalmoscopy: In IDDM, once a year after the first 5 years. In NIDDM, once a year after the first 2 years

Refer to ophthalmologist in case of: proliferations, maculopathy, impaired vision, or increased intraocular pressure

Indications for Consideration of Vitrectomy

If primary corpus vitreum bleeding does not clear up in 3 months
Recurrent corpus vitreum bleeding
Corpus vitreum cord fixed to retina
Traction amotio

Referral to an Institute for the Blind

Indications combine educational, occupational rehabilitation, psycho-social, and optical factors
The time when aid is needed varies and is not only related to a particular visual acuity or visual field limit

Hyperlipidaemia in Diabetes Mellitus

Recommendation for Lipid and Lipoprotein Levels

NIH Consensus[1]

Age (years)	Recommended cholesterol level (mmol/l)
<30	<4.6
>40	<5.2

Study group of the European Atherosclerosis Society[2]

	Recommended level (mmol/l)
Cholesterol	<5.2
Triglyceride	<2.3
HDL cholesterol	>0.9

---

[1] NIH Consensus Conference (1985) Lowering blood cholesterol to prevent heart disease. JAMA 253:2080–2086.

[2] Study Group of the European Atherosclerosis Society (1987) Strategies for the prevention of coronary heart disease: a policy statement of the European Atherosclerosis Society. Eur Heart J 8:77–88.

Calculation of Cholesterol Levels

VLDL = Very low density lipoproteins
LDL = Low-density lipoproteins
HDL = High-density lipoproteins
TG   = Triglyceride

VLDL cholesterol:

$$\frac{\text{Triglyceride}}{2.19} \text{ (presupposes that triglyeride} < 4 \text{ mmol/l)}$$

LDL cholesterol:

$$\text{Total cholesterol} - \left(\frac{\text{triglyceride}}{2.19} - \text{HDL cholesterol} \right)$$

Probable Sites of Action of Lipid-Lowering Drugs

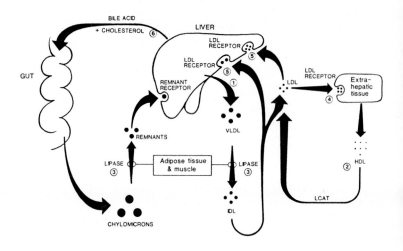

Model for plasma triglyceride and cholesterol transport in humans and schematic representation of the probable site of action of the most common lipid-lowering drugs:

1, Decrease in VLDL synthesis: fibrates, niacin
2, Increased synthesis of HDL: niacin, fibrates
3, Stimulation of lipoprotein lipase activity: fibrates
4, Increased number of LDL receptors: bile acid sequestrants, HMG-CoA reductase inhibitors, probucol?
5, Increased faecal excretion of bile acid sequestrants, probucol

LCAT, lecithin-cholesterol acyltransferase; *IDL,* intermediate-density lipoprotein

Approach to Diagnosis of Lipid Disorders

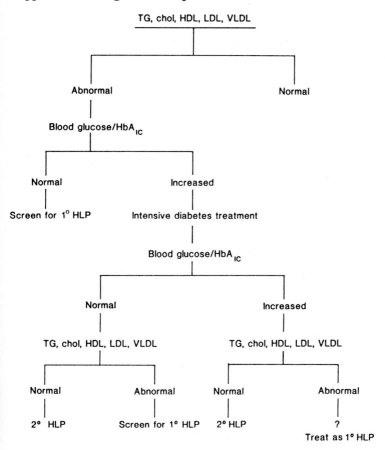

HLP, hyperlipoproteinaemia

Decision Process in Treatment of Lipid Disorders

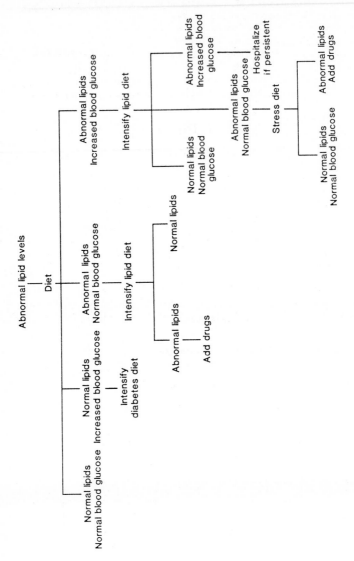

Types of Lipid/Lipoprotein Disorders

Lipid disorder	Lipoprotein abnormality
Chylomicronaemia syndrome	VLDL ↑ Chylomicrons ↑ HDL ↓
Endogenous hypertriglyceridaemia	VLDL ↑ HDL ↓
Combined hyperlipidaemia	VLDL ↑ LDL ↑
Dysbetalipoproteinaemia	Chylomicrons ↑ VLDL remnants ↑
Hypercholesterolaemia	LDL ↑
Hypoalphalipoproteinaemia	HDL ↓

Drugs Used in the Treatment of Lipid/Lipoprotein Disorders

Lipid disorder	Pharmacologic therapy	
	1st choice	2nd choice
Chylomicronaemia syndrome	Gemfibrozil	Niacin, clofibrate, bezafibrate
Endogenous hypertriglyceridaemia	Gemfibrozil	Niacin, clofibrate, bezafibrate
Combined hyperlipidaemia	HMG-CoA reductase inhibitors, niacin, gemfibrozil, colestipol, cholestyramine	Probucol
Dysbetalipoproteinaemia	HMG-CoA reductase inhibitors, clofibrate, bezafibrate	Gemfibrozil, niacin
Hypercholesterolaemia	HMG-CoA reductase inhibitors, colestipol, cholestyramine, niacin	Gemfibrozil, niacin

Prognosis and Cause of Death in Diabetic Patients[1]

Incidence of Complications After 40–50 Years with Insulin-Dependent Diabetes Mellitus

	%
Blindness/decreased vision	33
Myocardial infarction	20
Amputation	10
Nephropathy	33

Cause of Death in Diabetics

	IDDM (%)	NIDDM (%)
Nephropathy	33	10
Myocardial infarction	25	66

[1] Deckert T, Poulsen JE, Larsen M (1978) Prognosis of diabetics with diabetes onset before the age of 31. I: Survival, cause of death, and complications. Diabetologia 14:359–362.

111

Genetics of Diabetes

Diabetes and HLA

Prevalence of HLA type	(%)	
	IDDM	Controls
DR 3/3, DR 4/4, DR 3/4	90	60
DR 3/4	50	3

Risks for Insulin-Dependent Diabetes Mellitus

Population Risks

Overall	1/500
HLA-DR 3/3 or DR 4/4	1/150
HLA-DR 3/4	1/40

Relative Risks in Siblings

Overall	1/14
HLA haplotype shared with diabetic sibling	
0 haplotype shared	1/100
1 haplotype shared	1/20
2 haplotypes shared	1/6
2 haplotypes shared and DR 3/4	1/5–1/4

Risks for Offspring

Overall	1/25
Offspring of affected female	1/50–1/40
Offspring of affected male	1/20
Monozygotic twin of diabetic	1/3

Genetic Counselling[1]

Diabetes Risks

Risk person	Risk of acquiring diabetes (%)	
	Before 20 years of age	After 20 years of age
Siblings of a diabetic patient with start <20 years of age when parents are non-diabetic	5	5
Siblings of 2 diabetic patients with start <20 years of age when parents are non-diabetic	10	10
Siblings of a diabetic patient, one of the parents also diabetic, both with start <20 years of age	10	10

---

[1] Stevenson AC, Davison BCC (1975) Genetic counselling. Heinemann, London.

Person at risk	Risk of acquiring diabetes (%)	
	Before 20 years of age	After 20 years of age
Siblings of a diabetic patient with onset <20 years of age, one of the parents also diabetic but with onset >20 years of age	7	7
Siblings of a diabetic patient with onset <20 years of age, both parents also diabetic	20	20
Child of diabetic patient with onset <20 years of age (siblings non-diabetic)	10	(5)
Child of diabetic patient with onset >20 years of age (siblings non-diabetic)	5	3
Child of two diabetic patients with onset <20 years of age (siblings non-diabetic)	20	(10)
Child of two diabetic patients both with onset >20 years of age (siblings non-diabetic)	5	(3)

Diabetes Identity Cards

A. Insulin-Dependent

English. I am a diabetic having daily Insulin. If I am found ill please give me two tablespoons of sugar preferably in water. There should be sugar in my pocket or bag. If I am unconscious or do not recover please call a doctor or ambulance.

Dutch. Ik ben een suikerpatient en moet dagelijks insuline hebben. Als ik onwel word geef mij dan alstublieft twee eetlepels suiker opgelost in water. Er is suiker in mijn zak of tasje. Indien ik buiten kennis ben en neit bijkom wilt U dan alstublieft een doktor of een ziekenauto laten komen.

Finnish. Olen insuliinihoitoinen diabeetikko. Jos vaikutan sairaalta, antakaa minule kaksi ruokalusikallista sokeria mieluiten veteensekoitettuna. Taskussani tai laukussani pitäisi olla sokeria. Jos olen tajuton tai tilani ei kohene, kutsukaa lääkäri tai ambulanssi.

French. Je suis diabétique ayant besoin d'insuline quotidiennement. Si je me trouve mal donnez-moi, je vous prie, deux grandes cuillerées de sucre que je porte dans ma poche ou mon sac, avec de l'eau. Si je perds connaissance ou ne reviens pas a moi alertez, s'il vous plaît, un médicin ou une ambulance.

German. Ich bin Diabetiker und brauche täglich Insulin. Finden Sie mich krank, geben Sie mir bitte zwei Esslöffel Zucker in Wasser aufgelöst. Der Zucker befindet sich in meiner Tasche oder Handtasche. Finden Sie mich ohnmächtig, rufen Sie bitte einen Arzt oder einen Krankenwagen.

Italian. Sono un diabetico e ho bisogno di una dose giornaliera di insulina. Nel caso dovessi sentiemi male, prego di darmi due cucchiai di zucchero sciolti in acqua. Lo zucchero si trovera nelle mie tasche o nella mia borsa. Nel caso perdessi conoscenza o non dovessi rinvenire, si prega di chiamare un medico o un'ambulanza.

Norwegian. Jeg har sukkersyke og bruker daglig insulin. Hvis jeg blir funnet syk, vennligst gi meg to spiseskjeer sukker rørt i vann. Det er sukker i min lomme eller min veske. Hvis jeg er bevisstløs eller ikke våkner, vennligst tilkall lege eller sykebil.

Portuguese. Sou um doente diabético usando diaramente insulina. Se me encontrarem doente deêm-me faz favor duas colheres de sopa de açúcar em água. Encontrarào açúcar no meu bolso ou bolsa. Se me encontrarem inconsciente sem recuperaraçào, façam o favor de chamar um médico ou uma ambulância.

Spanish. Soy diabético y necesito insulina todos los dias. Si alguien me encontrara enfermo que me den, por favor, dos cucharadas de azúcar diluidas en agua. Encontrarán azúcar en uno de mis bolsillos o en mi saco. Si he perdido el conocimiento, o no me recupero, hagan el favor de llamar a un médico o a la ambulancia.

Swedish. Jag är diabetiker och tar dagligen insulin. Om Ni påträffar mig sjuk, var snäll och ge mig två matskedar socker i vatten. Det bör finnas socker i min ficka eller väska. Om jag är medvetslös eller inte tillfrisknar, var snäll och ring efter doktor eller ambulans.

8.8.   10/86

B. Oral Hypoglycaemic Agents

English. I am a diabetic taking tablets. If I am found ill please give me two tablespoons of sugar preferably in water. There should be sugar in my pocket or bag. If I am unconscious or do not recover please call a doctor or ambulance.

Dutch. Ik ben een suikerpatient die tabletten neemt. Als ik onwel word geef mij dan alstublieft twee eetlepels suiker opgelost in water. Er is suiker in mijn zak of tasje. Indien ik buiten kennis ben en neit bijkom wilt U dan alstublieft een doktor of een ziekenauto laten komen.

Finnish. Olen tablettihoitoinen diabeetikko. Jos vaikutan sairaalta, antakaa minule kaksi ruokalusikallista sokeria mieluiten veteensekoi-tettuna. Taskussani tai laukussani pitäisi olla sokeria. Jos olen tajuton tai tilani ei kohene, kutsukaa lääkäri tai ambulanssi.

French. Je suis diabétique et j'ai besoin de prendre des comprimés. Si je me trouve mal donnez-moi, je vous prie, deux grandes cuillerées de sucre que je porte dans ma poche ou mon sac, avec de l'eau. Si je perds connaissance ou ne reviens pas a moi alertez, s'il vous plaît, un médicin ou une ambulance.

German. Ich bin Diabetiker und nehme Tabletten. Wenn Sie mich krank finden, geben Sie mir bitte zwei Esslöffel Zucker in Wasser aufgelöst. Der Zucker befindet sich in meiner Tasche oder Handtasche. Wenn Sie mich ohnmächtig finden, rufen Sie bitte einen Arzt oder einen Krankenwagen.

Italian. Sono un Diabetico in cura con pastiglie. Nel caso dovessi sentiemi male, prego di darmi due cucchiai di zucchero sciolti in acqua. Lo zucchero si trovera nelle mie tasche o nella mia borsa. Nel caso perdessi conoscenza o non dovessi rinvenire, si prega di chiamare un medico o un'ambulanza.

Norwegian. Jeg har sukkersyke og tar tabletter. Hvis jeg blir funnet syk, vennligst gi meg to spiseskjeer sukker rørt i vann. Det er sukker i min lomme eller min veske. Hvis jeg er bevisstløs eller ikke våkner, vennligst tilkall lege eller sykebil.

Portuguese. Sou Diabético usando comprimidos. Se me encontra-rem doente deêm-me faz favor duas colheres de sopa de açúcar em água. Encontrarào açúcar no meu bolso ou bolsa. Se me encon-trarem inconsciente sem recuperaração, façam o favor de chamar um médico ou uma ambulância.

Spanish. Soy diabético y necesito tomar comprimidos. Si se me encontrara enfermo que me den, por favor, dos cucharadas de azúcar diluidas en agua. Encontrarán azúcar en uno de mis bolsillos o en un saquito. Si he perdido el conocimiento, o no me recupero, hagan el favor de llamar a un médico o a la ambulancia.

Swedish. Jag är diabetiker och tar tabletter. Om Ni påträffar mig sjuk, var snäll och ge mig två matskedar socker i vatten. Det bör finnas socker i min ficka eller väska. Om jag är medvetslös eller inte tillfriskar, var snäll och ring efter doktor eller ambulans.

10/86   8.8.1.

Index